Trudeau's MAiD Service

A Euthanasia Program for Canada

Trudeau's MAiD Service

A Euthanasia Program for Canada

David Cooke

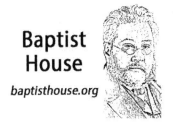

Baptist House

baptisthouse.org

Second Edition

Trudeau's MAiD Service:
A Euthanasia Program for Canada
Copyright © 2022 David T. E. S. Cooke

ISBN: 978-1-7774138-2-8

Published by Baptist House
Baker Brook, New Brunswick, Canada
baptisthouse.org

Cover Photograph by David Cooke
Notre-Dame-du-Rosaire Cemetery
Connors, New Brunswick, Canada, 2022

SOLI DEO GLORIA

DEDICATION

In memory of my mother,
who taught me by word and example
to stand up for what's right.

ACKNOWLEDGEMENT

With much thanks to my loving critic
and proof-reader – my wife.

THE LAW is there to protect us, so we are told. It maintains order, safeguards life, and defends our rights. But when we consider the current state of Canadian law, the words of Charles Dickens' Mr. Bumble jump to mind: "The law is an ass."

How else can we describe the advent of something called "Medical Assistance in Dying" (MAiD)? Here we have the *legal murder of a consenting victim.* How can such a horror ever become the law of the land?

And yet it has.

Canada has opened up a Pandora's box of death that only four other nations have dared to open before it.[1] And it will take an act of God to shut this box!

In 2015, the Supreme Court of Canada ruled (in Carter v. Canada) that "people who are grievously and irremediably ill" must be allowed to receive euthanasia.[2] A new "right to die" was invented out of thin air by nine judges, coaxed out of a twisted reinterpretation of our constitutional "right to life". This is something none of our Constitution's authors (in 1982), nor our founding fathers (in

1867), would ever have imagined.

Not only did this judicial fancy overturn all previous legal precedents, which had consistently denounced euthanasia, it discarded centuries of common law and common sense. Human life would no longer be unconditionally protected until its natural end. Those who are suffering could now be viewed differently – as *killable*.

Thus the cornerstone principle of human equality would be set aside as one human is granted the legal licence to destroy another human without repercussion.

The ancient biblical precepts that undergird our legal system and impart the blessing of God to our nation were cast aside in this ruling. And not one judge raised a voice of dissent!

In particular, the Sixth Commandment, "Thou shalt not kill,"[3] had inexplicably become, "Thou shalt kill"; for this fabricated "right to die" requires someone to *kill,* and someone to *be killed*.

The Liberal government of Justin Trudeau eagerly accepted the Supreme Court's revolutionary ruling and quickly enacted Bill C-14 into law on June 17, 2016. This law created an exception in our Criminal Code for what was hitherto recognized as "first degree murder" (i.e. a "planned and deliberate" killing).

Under Bill C-14, if a terminally ill adult gave his consent, and his death was thought to be "reasonably foreseeable", he could be legally murdered or assisted in his own suicide. This law also carved out exceptions for participating doctors, nurses, and pharmacists who, previously, would have been classified as *murderers, accessories to murder,* and *abettors of suicide* – some of the most serious criminal offences known to man.

The Minister of Justice at that time, Jody Wilson-Raybould, stunningly admitted that "medical assistance in dying is exceptional because, from a criminal law perspective, it is a situation where one person actively and knowingly participates in the death of another. *We criminalize and strongly condemn this conduct in all other circumstances."*[4]

With the introduction of legal euthanasia, a new euphemism was coined: "Medical Assistance in Dying" or MAiD. Here is a slogan that must have been birthed by a million-dollar advertising agency!

In order to assuage the nation's moral sensibilities, this sterilized form of medical murder was dressed in the garb of a kindly servant-girl, ready to lend a "helping hand" at no charge. It just so happens that hand bears a syringe with a lethal injection.

However, even this radical liberalization of killing was not enough for some. David Lametti, who would later take over as Minister of Justice, insisted that Bill C-14 was too restrictive.[5] Thus, after passage, the Trudeau government tasked the Council of Canadian Academies with researching three gruesome concepts: *euthanasia for children, euthanasia for those who are incompetent,* and *euthanasia for the mentally ill.*[6]

In late 2018, MAiD proponents at Toronto's Hospital for Sick Children released their own recommendation. They declared that the murder of suffering children is perfectly "ethical", even if parents object, as long as the child is deemed to have "consented".[7]

In September 2019, a single Quebec judge, Christine Baudouin, ruled that euthanasia must not be limited to patients whose deaths are "reasonably foreseeable", decreeing that Bill C-14's provisions *must* be expanded. Not only those who are terminal, but those who are disabled should qualify, even if they are not actually dying, according to the judge.

Taking this as an excuse to allow more killing, the Trudeau government made this ruling the law of the land with the passage of Bill C-7 in 2021. This took place *before* the promised statutory review, which was supposed to study the impact of the law and correct any errors.

Under Bill C-7, Canada now permits those with disabilities, even if they are otherwise healthy and functional, to receive MAiD. If their disability is considered "serious" and "incurable", if they are in an "advanced state of irreversible decline in capability" in some area, and if they believe they experience "physical or psychological suffering that is intolerable," then MAiD will be approved.[8]

They will be murdered.

Of course, there are no actual definitions for all of these criteria. Everything is totally subjective, effectively allowing anyone with any disability or disease to qualify.

For example, when a 51-year-old woman with serious environmental allergies said she could not cope with the smells coming from her neighbours' apartments, she was approved for MAiD. Instead of providing her with new housing, her execution was carried out on February 22, 2022.[9]

It has become that easy to kill and be killed!

Bill C-7 also allows for those who are mentally ill to secure a hastened death under these same nebulous criteria, starting on March 17, 2023. This means that all our efforts at suicide prevention are about to be turned on their head.

Stopping people from killing themselves will soon be seen as interfering with their rights.

Even if there is an effective treatment or cure available to those who are depressed, disabled, or diseased, under Trudeau's euthanasia program, these troubled souls *shall not* be denied a lethal injection, if they request one. The would-be victim is under *no* obligation to seek healing over killing. He need not be given any incentive or encouragement to live.

The choice of death is so "sacred" that it must trump the option of recovery. The *new crime* will not be *murder,* but *interfering with murder.*

The Liberal government is exerting every effort to make killing as accessible and easy as possible for more and more Canadians. And for those whose deaths are deemed "reasonably foreseeable", the government is so accommodating that it now permits them to be executed the *same day* – on the spot – without any opportunity to repent and without any urging to reconsider.

It is worth noting that we do not treat mass-murderers with such inhumanity! Capital punishment was outlawed in Canada in 1976 out of concern for human rights, particularly the right to life. We were told that those who kill must not be killed; but now killing with consent is somehow justified.

It has become fashionable to allow people to lose all hope, abandon their will to live, and be killed.

And while the law provides for a last-second opt-out for those who "by words, sounds or gestures" happen to experience a change of heart, the law also states that if the "words, sounds or gestures" are deemed "involuntary", the murder will go ahead as scheduled. Thus even a flickering will to live can be snuffed out by our killing professionals!

In 2022, a new proposal was made in the Senate under Bill S-248, which would allow for *future guaranteed killing* as an added option. That means if one should experience dementia, a loss of consciousness, or fall into a coma at some future date, one can be killed without the need for immediate consent.

By signing an *advanced directive,* you can agree to MAiD years ahead of time, not knowing what will actually happen or how your beliefs and values might change over time. Under this frightening concept, a doctor or nurse – who is usually a complete stranger – will decide your fate for you.

It seems that we are well on our way to the unthinkable – what no one is willing to admit – "euthanasia on demand".

Following our nation's track-record on elective abortion, which is permitted through all nine months of pregnancy and "on demand", we may eventually permit elective euthanasia at any age, for any reason, or *for no reason at all*. There appears to be a devilish logic to this.

Certainly, with euthanasia deaths growing year by year, and with very few objections being voiced in mainstream media and academia, we should expect the legal restraints to loosen further. The more people opt for MAiD, the more the government thinks it can justify expanding MAiD.

According to the latest statistics, euthanasia deaths have increased significantly every single year. The total number of Canadians who were euthanized from 2016 to the end of 2021 was 31,664. That is roughly the entire population of Stratford, Ontario. Can you imagine the city of Stratford wiped off the face of the earth? And the Trudeau government is pleased.

But what are the dangers of legalized

euthanasia? Why is the "right to die" (i.e. to die an unnatural and hastened death) such a concern?

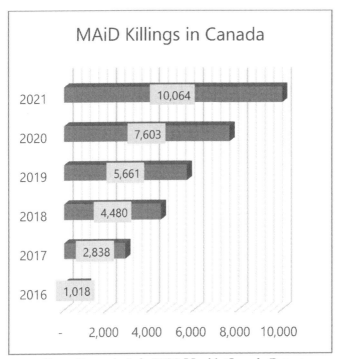

MAiD Killings in Canada

Year	Count
2021	10,064
2020	7,603
2019	5,661
2018	4,480
2017	2,838
2016	1,018

- 2,000 4,000 6,000 8,000 10,000

Above: From the July 2022 Health Canada Report, "Medical Assistance in Dying in Canada 2021", p. 18.[10]

For one, consider the economics of this so-called "treatment option". As a cost-cutting measure, MAiD is an instant boon to our socialized healthcare system. That's why doctors are being pushed to offer it, and patients are being pressured to accept it. One lethal injection saves time and money over every other course of action.

This sets up the system to favour killing, especially with an ageing population.[11] Perhaps that is why we are hearing more accounts of Canadians being propositioned with MAiD by medical staff and government bureaucrats.[12]

Also, euthanasia not only destroys human life, it destroys the value of human life. Why bother fighting for your life if an "easy death" is available? If it is legal (and you are told it is your "right") then you might just think it is for the best, especially if it comes "doctor recommended" and helps save our fragile healthcare system.

Human life becomes disposable instead of sacrosanct. Our dignity is discarded instead of defended to life's natural end.

And what happens when the "right to die" becomes a "duty to die"? Feelings of "being a burden" are common among the sick, elderly, disabled, and mentally ill. Many will think they have no choice.

Furthermore, there will always be those "loved ones" who are more eager for Granny's inheritance than for Granny's presence, who will push and push until Granny gives in and requests MAiD. That is what human greed does.

Statistics from last year reveal that 3% of those

who were murdered by MAiD gave their consent because of feelings like "anxiety" or "fear". A total of 17.3% did so because of feelings of "isolation or loneliness". A whopping 54.3% felt that they had lost their "dignity".[13]

But these are mere *perceptions* and *emotions,* all of which could easily be remedied with improved healthcare, better homecare options, more caring and compassionate staff, and the offer of spiritual and psychological guidance. People crave hope, meaning, and love in their hour of need, but MAiD offers none of these.

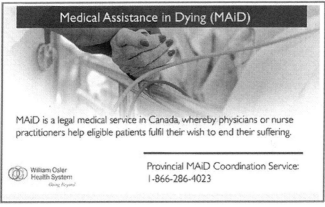

Above: An advertisement for MAiD in an Ontario hospital encourages patients to consent to be killed.

And what about mistakes? Mistakes have been known to happen in healthcare. What if a patient's wishes are misunderstood? What if a person changes his mind but cannot express that change of mind – or his expressions of refusal are deemed "involuntary"?

Or what if that lethal injection is administered to the wrong patient in the wrong bed?

It will be easy to brush these mistakes under the rug when the victims are no longer around to complain or file a lawsuit!

But most importantly, *have we counted the spiritual cost?* For surely there is a cost to throwing God's gift of life back in His face! Surely there is a cost when we, as a society, allow some to play God while we allow others to be victimized.

In the Scriptures, Moses gives us this biblical precept: "I have set before you life and death, blessing and cursing; therefore choose life, that both you and your descendants may live."[14]

The choice of life is a blessing; the choice of death is a curse – both individually and societally.

We would do well to heed the lessons of history when it comes to toying with legalized murder.

In 1920, an academic paper was published by two German scholars (Binding and Hoche). They explored a new concept called "life unworthy of life". Their research led to the Nazi's "Aktion T4" program in 1939. After the public was sold on the concept, T4 provided legal euthanasia for disabled children and adults as "an act of mercy".

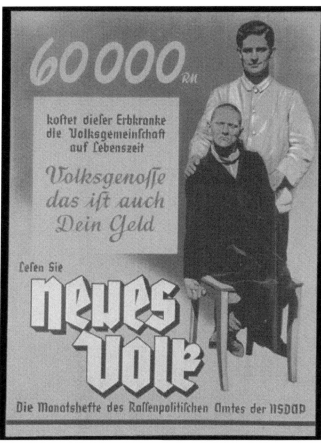

Above: A 1938 poster promoting the Nazi euthanasia program as a merciful, cost-saving treatment option. It reads: "This hereditary defective costs the Volk community 60,000 RM over his lifetime. German comrade, that is your money."

This program, in the months and years that

followed, formed the basis for the Holocaust, which executed millions who were not only deemed medically "unfit", but socially, politically, and racially "unfit".

Who is to say that Canada's present euthanasia experiment will not yield similar results if allowed to run its *unnatural* course? As history proves, once men believe they can play God, it is easy to go from one form of killing to another.

In Canada, we began with killing preborn children through legalized elective abortion. Now we kill terminally ill and disabled adults. In 2023 we will kill depressed adults.

Who will be next? Sick children? Troubled teens? Homeless people? The unemployed? Dementia patients? What about those deemed politically "unfit"? What about those of a particular race or religion?

Who is to say some future government could not mandate this procedure for certain groups of *unacceptable* citizens? If two years of COVID-19 have taught us anything, it is our government's willingness to impose medical interventions and coerce consent in the midst of a perceived crisis.

What future crisis might herald a call for mandatory MAiD?

We are playing a very dangerous game. With the advent of legal euthanasia, our medical professionals are becoming calloused *grim reapers,* while our hospitals are becoming *butcher shops* – especially when their victims are also organ donors. Do we imagine anyone will be safe with such a murderous cancer growing and metastasizing within our healthcare system?

MAiD represents a fundamental perversion of human rights and medical ethics. This must not be allowed to continue.

In the Hippocratic Oath, the standard of medical conduct since the 5th century BC, doctors pledge: "I will not give a lethal drug to anyone if I am asked, nor will I advise such a plan."

According to the World Medical Association (WMA) in their 2019 policy statement: "The WMA reiterates its strong commitment to the principles of medical ethics and that utmost respect has to be maintained for human life. Therefore, the WMA is firmly opposed to euthanasia and physician-assisted suicide."

With the advent of Trudeau's "MAiD service" in Canada, a deadly Pandora's box has been opened, and we are loath to see what comes out next!

Our only hope is to turn back to the One who

is the true Lawgiver and Author of Life, Almighty God, through His Son, our Lord Jesus Christ.

For the protection of every human life in Canada, the Sixth Commandment must be reclaimed – "Thou shalt not kill."

No human can be permitted to kill any other innocent human – *ever*.

No human is killable. Every human is equal!

Therefore, with a message of hope, meaning, and love for those who are suffering, as we strive to provide them with the genuine support and care they need, let us choose life and blessing once again for our nation. Let us end this asinine euthanasia law and put a stop to Trudeau's MAiD service.[15]

As God promises in the Scriptures: "If My people who are called by My name will humble themselves, and pray and seek My face, and turn from their wicked ways, then I will hear from heaven, and will forgive their sin and heal their land."[16]

NOTES

[1] Netherlands (2002), Belgium (2002), Luxembourg (2009), and Colombia (2014) were the first nations to legalize euthanasia.

[2] https://www.canlii.org/en/ca/scc/doc/2015/2015scc5/2015scc5.html

[3] Exodus 20:13 (KJV).

[4] *Emphasis added.* Hansard, House of Commons, Parliament of Canada, 62 (May 31, 2016).

[5] http://alexschadenberg.blogspot.com/2019/02/ canadian-media-promotes-euthanasia.html

[6] https://www.lifesitenews.com/opinion/canada-may-make-mentally-ill-subject-to-assisted-suicide

[7] http://jme.bmj.com/content/45/1/60

[8] Criminal Code of Canada, Section 241.2(2).

[9] https://www.ctvnews.ca/health/woman-with-chemical-sensitivities-chose-medically-assisted-death-after-failed-bid-to-get-better-housing-1.5860579

[10] https://www.canada.ca/content/dam/hc-sc/documents/services/medical-assistance-dying/annual-report-2021/annual-report-2021.pdf

[11] https://census.gc.ca/census-recensement/2021/as-sa/98-200-X/2021003/98-200-X2021003-eng.cfm

[12] https://globalnews.ca/news/9061709/veteran-medical-assisted-death-canada/ and https://www.ctvnews.ca/health/chronically-ill-man-releases-audio-of-hospital-staff-offering-assisted-death-1.4038841

[13] "Medical Assistance in Dying in Canada 2021", Health Canada (July 2022), p. 26.

[14] Deuteronomy 30:19 (NKJV).

[15] For help and resources to combat the expansion of euthanasia in Canada, please contact Campaign Life Coalition (http://campaignlifecoalition.com) or Euthanasia Prevention Coalition (http://epcc.ca).

[16] 2 Chronicles 7:14 (NKJV).

APPENDIX

The following article was published in the New York Times on October 7, 1933, unveiling the initial plans for a Nazi euthanasia program. This program was eventually launched in 1939 as "Aktion T4", which prepared the way for the Holocaust.

Notice how the Nazi program emphasized the need for consent, much like MAiD does. Also notice the claim that killing is somehow "in the interests of true humanity", which is often how MAiD is characterized.

Ultimately, MAiD, like T4, goes wrong by measuring the worth of a human life in its limited value to the State, not in its immeasurable value to God.

Nazis Plan to Kill Incurables to End Pain; German Religious Groups Oppose Move
By The Associated Press

BERLIN, Oct. 7.—The Ministry of Justice in a detailed memorandum explaining the Nazi aims regarding the German penal code today announced its intention to authorize physicians to end the sufferings of incurable patients.

The memorandum, still lacking the force of law, proposed that "it shall be made possible for physicians to end the tortures of incurable patients, upon request, in the interests of true humanity."

This proposed legal recognition of euthanasia—the act of providing a painless and peaceful death—raised a number of fundamental problems of a religious, scientific and legal nature.

The Catholic newspaper Germania hastened to observe:

"The Catholic faith binds the conscience of its followers not to accept this method of shortening the sufferings of incurables who are tormented by pain."

In Lutheran circles, too, life is regarded as something that God alone can take.

A large section of the German people, it was expected in some interested circles, might ignore the provisions for euthanasia, which overnight has become a widely-discussed word in the Reich.

In medical circles the question was raised as to just when a man is incurable and when his life should be ended.

According to the present plans of the Ministry of Justice, incurability would be determined not only by the attending physician, but also by two official doctors who would carefully trace the history of the case and personally examine the patient.

In insisting that euthanasia shall be permissible only if the accredited attending physician is backed by two experts who so advise, the Ministry believes a guarantee is given that no life still valuable to the State will be wantonly destroyed.

The legal question of who may request the application of euthanasia has not been definitely solved. The Ministry merely has proposed that either the patient himself shall "expressly and earnestly" ask it, or "in case the patient no longer is able to express his desire, his nearer relatives, acting from motives that do not contravene morals, so request."

ABOUT THE AUTHOR

David Cooke graduated from Queen's University with a Bachelor of Arts, and from Toronto Baptist Seminary with a Master of Divinity. He served as a church pastor in Ontario, Canada, and as a missionary teacher in Honduras. He presently serves with Campaign Life Coalition, and also does itinerant preaching and teaching. He is married and has two children.

Manufactured by Amazon.ca
Bolton, ON